NUTRIENT AGAINST CANCER

Many scientific studies confirm that the nutrient D-glucarate is one of the major detoxifying components in fruits and vegetables. Calcium D-glucarate, now available as a supplement, has been shown to be effective in reducing the risk of various cancers by eliminating toxins from the body. State-of-the-art research confirms the potential of this nutrient as a major player in cancer risk reduction.

Thomas J. Slaga received his Ph.D. degree in physiology and biochemistry from the University of Arkansas Medical Center in 1969. From 1968 to 1971, he carried out postdoctoral work at the McArdle Laboratory for Cancer Research at the University of Wisconsin. He then moved to Seattle where he held positions at the Pacific Northwest Research Foundation, the Fred Hutchinson Cancer Research Center, and the University of Washington. He also spent several years as a group leader at the Oak Ridge National Laboratory. From 1982 to 1997, Dr. Slaga served as the director of the Science Park–Research Division of the University of Texas M. D. Anderson Cancer Center. Under his direction, the Science Park Division earned a reputation for research excellence in carcinogenesis and in cancer prevention. In August of 1997, Dr. Slaga was recruited to the AMC Cancer Research Center in Denver where he became chair of the Center for Cancer Causation and Prevention; in mid-1998, he accepted the position of executive vice president for research on the AMC campus.

Dr. Slaga's research focuses on determining the critical cellular and molecular mechanisms in epithelial tissues during carcinogenesis. These studies are being investigated primarily in mouse skin, a model where carcinogenesis can occur by a multistage process. Currently, Dr. Slaga is focusing on the importance of specific protein changes, loss of the glucocorticoid receptor and/or function, and the importance of genetic instability in this multistage process.

Dr. Slaga has authored or co-authored more than 375 journal articles, book chapters, and reviews. He is widely recognized for his outstanding scientific contributions in the area of multistage carcinogenesis. In addition, Dr. Slaga has edited more than twenty books dealing with cancer causation and prevention. He also serves on numerous editorial boards, study sections, scientific advisory boards, and committees. Dr. Slaga has been the editor-in-chief of *Molecular Carcinogenesis* since its inception.

Judi Quilici-Timmcke has master degrees in dietetics and exercise physiology. She was in private practice as a clinical nutritionist for twelve years in Colorado, including two-and-a-half years for the University of Colorado at Boulder's Human Performance Lab. She taught nutrition, biology, anatomy, and physiology at the college level for four years and has lectured on nutrition for various associations around the country. She taught nutrition to low-income populations for the mayor's office in Chicago and on Indian reservations for the Wisconsin Department of Health and Human Services. She has also been a consultant for the NCAA and the President's Council on Physical Fitness, where she evaluated low-income youth sports and lunch programs around the United States. She presently writes literature reviews about dietary supplements, writes scientific reports, formulates products for the dietary supplement industry, and presents scientific research on television and radio programs nationally. She writes nutrition articles for magazines and is the author of another Good Health Guide entitled *New Nutrients Against Cancer*. She is also a member of the Corporate Alliance for Integrative Medicine and the American Dietetic Association.

D-Glucarate:
A Nutrient
Against Cancer

A new breakthrough in cancer
research: D-glucarate helps remove
toxins and carcinogens
from the body

by Thomas J. Slaga, Ph.D.
and Judi Quilici-Timmcke, M.S.

KEATS PUBLISHING

LOS ANGELES

NTC/Contemporary Publishing Group

D-Glucarate: A Nutrient Against Cancer is intended solely for informational and educational purposes and not as medical advice. Please consult a health care professional if you have questions about your health.

D-GLUCARATE: A NUTRIENT AGAINST CANCER

Published by Keats
A division of NTC/Contemporary Publishing Group, Inc.
4255 West Touhy Avenue, Lincolnwood (Chicago), Illinois 60646-1975 U.S.A.
International Standard Book Number: 0-87983-952-X

15 16 17 18 19 20 QVS/QVS 20 19 18 17 16

Contents

WHAT IS CANCER?

Although there has been great progress in the last few decades in cancer research, there is still much that is not known. The exact cause of cancer is not completely understood, but we now have a greater appreciation of how our environment can contribute to the development of cancer. It has become very clear that diet plays an important role in cancer, and that risk reduction is probably our best chance of reducing cancer rates. In this Good Health Guide, we will discuss a promising supplement, calcium D-glucarate, that has been shown in numerous studies to reduce the risk of cancer with no known side effects. But before we discuss calcium D-glucarate, let's review some important concepts about cancer.

Many complicated changes exist in cancer cells compared with normal cells. Cancer cells undergo a process called *de-differentiation*. This means our cells change so that they no longer work together and instead become more independent. It has been known since the 1940s that de-differentiation results in cells that are more primitive in their appearance and function compared with normal functioning cells. De-differentiation is a complicated process. Many factors within the cells become different. Cancer cells typically use less oxygen in their energy production and instead tend to use a process called *fermentation*. You have probably heard of fermentation before. For example, it is used to make alcohol from yeast. In this process, glucose is metabolized for energy *anaerobically* (without oxygen) by yeast, with alcohol the resulting by-product. In cancer cells a similar process takes place, but the product of the anaerobic metabolism is called *lactate*. Bacteria are organisms that also use fermentation to make energy. So one concept that has emerged in cancer research is that cancer cells appear to be more like primitive bacterial cells, and their energy metabolism partially changes to a more primitive form.

There are other changes in our cells that are associated with cancer. Changes or *mutations* in our DNA are closely linked with cancer. DNA stands for *deoxyribonucleic acid*. DNA contains all the hereditary information in our cells. Most DNA exists in the *nucleus*, but some is also found in the *mitochondria*. The mitochondria are the *cellular organelles* that produce energy to drive the chemical reactions that sustain life. *Genes* are small pieces of DNA that give the cells the message to produce a specific protein. Proteins are the large molecules that perform most of the work in our bodies. *Oncogenes* are genes that are associated with some forms of cancer. Other genes known to be important in cancer are the tumor suppressor genes and the genes that regulate cell death, a natural process that eliminates old or dysfuntional cells in our body.

One of the most important questions in cancer research is why the cells change. Any process which stops the de-differentiation of cells will undoubtably be very beneficial for cancer treatment and risk reduction. Calcium D-glucarate has properties that suggest it may be useful in stopping the de-differentiation of cells by removing toxins and carcinogens. We will focus on calcium D-glucarate research in a later section. There is direct evidence that many different environmental situations can cause cells to de-differentiate into cancer cells. We will discuss some of the environmental factors in the next section.

Most cancers exist in the form of tumors. Tumors can be either benign or malignant. Benign tumors are not really cancer since they do not grow uncontrollably. Usually, benign tumors are not a threat to life unless they arise in a vital organ, such as the brain. But benign tumors have been known to progress to malignancy. Malignant tumors are cancerous since they grow rapidly and also affect adjacent tissues. Cancer cells can also spread, or *metastasize*, to other parts of the body through the bloodstream or lymphatic system.

Cancer is able to affect virtually every part of the body, and can be divided into at least the following categories: *carcinomas, sarcomas, myelomas, lymphomas, leukemias, neuroblastomas,* and *gliomas*. Cancer is defined by three different stages: *initiation, promotion,* and *progression.* Let's take a look at how we specifically define these stages. Initiation is the stage in which some fundamental process takes place at the cellular level to cause the de-differentiation process to begin. This change can occur many years before the harmful effects of cancer become evident. In the promotion stage, cancer cells begin to multiply rapidly and tumors begin to grow in size. In the last stage, progression, cancer cells are no longer localized in one tissue. They metastasize to other parts of the body. It is during this stage that cancer is often fatal.

In the United States, skin, lung, colon, breast, and prostate are the major cancers. The number of new cases of cancer in the United States is increasing each year. People of all ages get cancer; however, middle-aged and elderly people are most often affected. Skin cancer is the most common type of cancer in both men and women. Prostate cancer is the second most common in men, and breast cancer is the second most common in women. Lung cancer is still the leading cause of cancer deaths in both men and women in the United States. Brain cancer and leukemia are the most common cancers found in children and young adults.

WHAT CAUSES CANCER?

Cancers develop gradually as a result of a complex interaction of factors related to heredity, environment, lifestyle, and diet.[1,2,3] Table 1 summarizes some of these factors. Cancer scientists have identified many risk factors that increase the chances of an individual developing cancer. Based on scientific estimates, approximately 80 percent of all cancers are related to the use of tobacco products, to what we eat and drink, to exposure to sunlight and ionizing radiation, and to exposure to cancer-causing chemicals and agents found in the environment and the workplace.[4] It seems that some people are more sensitive than others to various factors that cause cancer. However, lifestyle factors account for most cancer risk: sun exposure, tobacco use, eating habits, and alcohol consumption. Table 2 shows estimated percentages of the leading possible causes of cancer.

ARE THERE RISKS WE CAN AVOID?

You can help protect yourself from developing cancer by choosing a lifestyle that eliminates certain risks. Many cancers are linked to the following factors that an individual can control.

Tobacco Use

Probably the strongest evidence linking cancer to a lifestyle choice is smoking and other uses of tobacco. These have been directly linked to cancer.[6,7] These practices have also been linked to other degenerative diseases such as heart disease, diseases of the circulatory system, emphysema, and chronic bronchitis.[6,7] Table 3 summarizes tobacco-related diseases.

Table 1
Factors Associated with Cancer

Environmental Factors	Lifestyle Factors	Heredity Factors
Chemicals	Smoking	Oncogenes
Radiation	Tobacco and alcohol	Tumor suppressor genes
Viruses	Diet and nutrition	
Physical agents (asbestos)	Total calories	
	Low fiber	
	Vitamin and mineral deficiencies	
	Preparation and cooking of foods	

Table 2
Estimated Percentage of Cancer Deaths Attributable to Various Factors

Factors	Percentage
Diet	35
Tobacco	30
Reproductive/sexual behavior	7
Occupation	4
Alcohol	3
Ultraviolet radiation	3
Pollution	2
Industrial products	<1
Food additives	1
Medicine/medical products	1

Source: Percentages from Doll and Peto, 1981, and Mynder and Gori, 1977.

Table 3
Health Concerns Directly Linked to Cigarette Smoking and Tobacco Products

- Cancer
- Cardiovascular disease
- Emphysema
- Chronic bronchitis
- Immune dysfunction
- Premature aging

Cigarette smoking is responsible for approximately 30 percent of all cancer deaths. The risk of developing lung cancer is ten times greater for smokers than for non-smokers. Of course, the degree of risk from smoking depends on the number and type of cigarettes smoked, the length of time an individual has smoked, and how deeply the the smoke is inhaled. The 1982 Surgeon General's Report labeled cigarette smoking "the single major cause of cancer deaths in the United States," a statement that is still accurate in 1999. Cigarette smoking and the use of other tobacco products are a major cause of cancers of the lung, the mouth, the larynx, and the esophagus. The use of these products also contributes

D-GLUCARATE: A NUTRIENT AGAINST CANCER / 13

significantly to cancers of the bladder, kidney, and pancreas. In addition, research studies have found an association between tobacco use and leukemias, breast, and prostate cancers.

A number of substances in cigarette smoke are both toxic and carcinogenic. Some of these are called *co-carcinogens*, which means that, when combined with other substances, they may produce cancerous cells. Also of concern are *cancer promoters*, so named because once cancer cells start to grow, cancer promoters cause the cancerous cells to multiply even faster. In general, there are many toxic, carcinogenic, co-carcinogenic and tumor-promoting agents in cigarette smoke and tobacco products.[6,7] In addition to the harmful substances in cigarette smoke and tobacco products, *free radicals* are formed, which have also been implicated in many degenerative diseases. We will discuss free radicals in more detail later. There are approximately four thousand currently known harmful substances in tobacco products. Table 4 summarizes the dangerous chemicals and gases found in cigarette smoke and other tobacco products.

Table 4
Some of the More Than 4,000 Dangerous and Carcinogenic Chemicals Found in Cigarette and Tobacco Products

• Glycols	• Hydrogen cyanide
• Alcohols	• Nitrogen oxide
• Aldehydes	• Carbon monoxide
• Ketones	• Radioactive elements
• Alkaloids	• Carcinogens
• Aliphatic hydrocarbons	• Tumor promoters
• Aromatic hydrocarbons	• Co-carcinogens
• Phenols	

Since it is clear that tobacco products contain many powerful carcinogens, the wisest choice is to stop using them. Diets high in fruits and vegetables have been associated with a decreased risk of acquiring tobacco- and smoking-related diseases, including cancer, in both smokers and ex-smokers.[8,9] Animal studies and *epidemiological* studies (comparative studies of populations and lifestyles) show that a variety of vitamins, minerals, antioxidants, and related *phytochemicals* (chemicals from plants) decrease the harmful effects of tobacco products.[8,10,11,12] As we will show later, D-glucarate, found naturally in fruits and vegetables, protects against cancer. Table 5 summarizes various classes of phytochemicals with cancer prevention properties.

Table 5
Classes of Phytochemicals with Cancer Prevention Properties

- D-glucarate and derivatives
- Flavonoids
- Isoflavones
- Polyphenols
- Terpenoids
- Indoles
- Isothiocyanates
- Organosulfides
- Tanins

Diet

There is extensive scientific agreement that what we consume will affect our chances of developing cancer. Since it is estimated that 35 percent of cancers are directly affected by diet and nutrition, it is possible that cancer could be prevented by selecting a diet thought to minimize cancer risk. There are more than two hundred epidemiological studies that suggest a diet high in fruits and vegetables may lead to a decrease in cancer.[9]

A tremendous amount of research suggests that reducing our total number of calories from carbohydrates, proteins, and fats may lead to reduced risk of cancer. In animal experiments, a 30 percent reduction in calories significantly decreased many induced and spontaneous cancers. Some scientists believe there is a link between high polyunsaturated fats in the diet (such as corn oil, margarine, and vegetable cooking oils) and some cancers, especially those of the breast, colon, endometrium, and prostate.[1]

Eating large amounts of smoked, cured, and pickled foods has been linked to esophagus and stomach cancer. A relationship has also been found between vitamin deficiencies and certain cancers, including liver, skin, and lung

Table 6
Relationships Between Diet and Cancer Risk

Probable Causative Agents	Type of Cancer
• Excess total calories	• *All* cancers
• Excess polyunsaturated fat	• Prostate, breast, colon, rectum, stomach, pancreas, ovary
• Excess alcohol	• Esophagus, mouth, head and neck, lip, stomach, liver, colon, rectum
• Selenium deficiency	• Many cancers
• Iron deficiency	• Stomach and esophagus
• Iodine deficiency	• Thyroid
• Excess smoked meat or fish, excess charcoal-broiled meat, pickled products	• Stomach and esophagus

cancer. In addition, mineral deficiencies of selenium, iodine, and iron may be related to cancers of the stomach, thyroid, esophagus, breast, and prostate. Table 6 summarizes the relationships between diet and cancer risk.

Sunlight and Radiation
Skin cancer is the most common cancer in the United States.[15,16] It is well known that repeated exposure to sunlight (ultraviolet radiation) increases the risk of acquiring both melanoma and non-melanoma skin cancer, especially if you have fair skin or freckle easily. Although some environmental chemicals may contribute to the *development* of skin cancer, ultraviolet radiation from the sun is the primary *cause* of skin cancer. In addition, ultraviolet radiation from other sources, such as sunlamps and tanning booths, can cause extensive damage to the skin, which may lead to skin cancer.

Protective clothing, such as a broad-brimmed hat and long-sleeved garments, can help block out the sun's harmful rays. Sunscreens can also be used to help protect exposed areas; such products must have a Sun Protection Factor (SPF) of at least 15, and contain both ultraviolet A and B absorbers. Our atmosphere's ozone layer provides protection against ultraviolet C radiation, but if the ozone layer continues to diminish, it may become necessary to provide protection against ultraviolet C as well. Exposure to large amounts of radiation from X rays has been shown to increase the risk of cancer.[15] However, the X rays typically used for medical and dental diagnoses expose you to very little radiation, and generally the benefits outweigh the risks. To safeguard your health, it is advisable to avoid unnecessary X rays, and to insist upon shielding the areas of your body not requiring X rays for diagnostic purposes. There is also evidence that selenium supplementation may reduce the risk of developing skin cancer.

Alcohol
Drinking large quantities of alcohol increases the risk of cancers of the mouth, throat, esophagus, and liver. One to two drinks of alcohol per day and no more than ten drinks per week is considered moderate drinking for men. Among women, one drink per day and a maximum of eight drinks per week is considered moderate. Moderate consumption may actually lead to a decrease in cancer, although additional research will be necessary to establish such guidelines. However, people who smoke cigarettes and drink excessive amounts of alcohol have a much higher incidence of cancers of the mouth and the esophagus.

Industrial Chemicals and Agents
Exposure to numerous environmental substances found in the workplace, such as metals, dust, and chemicals, can increase the incidence of certain cancers.[15] Benzene, benzidine, vinyl chloride, asbestos, uranium, radon, nickel, and cadmium are examples of cancer-causing agents sometimes found in the workplace.[5] Industrial agents can cause damage by acting alone or in conjunction with other cancer-causing agents, found either in the workplace or in cigarette smoke. For example, the inhalation of asbestos fibers increases the risk of lung disease, which can be further compounded if an individual smokes cigarettes.[15] Uranium mine workers who smoke also have an especially high risk of lung cancer.

Some industrial chemicals are dangerous if inhaled in high concentrations in areas that are not well ventilated. It is a good practice to avoid exposure to large amounts of household solvent cleaners, cleaning fluids, and petroleum products. You should be very careful when handling garden and lawn chemicals, and take necessary precautions against inhaling, ingesting, or spilling them on your skin. All of these exposures can increase your risk of cancer.

In summary, there are many cancer risk factors that you can control. Table 7 shows ways to significantly reduce your cancer risk.

Table 7
Ways to Reduce Cancer Risk

- Diet
    - Reduce calorie intake from all sources
    - Reduce percentage of calories from polyunsaturated fats
    - Increase fruit and vegetable consumption
    - Add vitamins, minerals, and phytochemical supplements
- Reduce or eliminate tobacco use
- Limit sunlight exposure
- Limit alcohol consumption

DETOXIFICATION

THE IMPORTANCE OF DETOXIFICATION

The term toxicity describes a condition that arises from an excessive concentration of harmful agents. The human body rids itself of toxins by a mechanism called *detoxification*. However, this removal of toxic substances depends on many factors, including genetics, poor diet, and/or disease. Our body defends itself by detoxifying harmful substances that are made in the body, that invade from our environment, or that are found in our diet. If a substance is not used for a specific purpose, such as building tissue or fuel for energy, that substance may be eliminated by the detoxification pathway. During detoxification, the body metabolizes these substances. This is accomplished by using chemical reactions that make the toxins more soluble in water. The toxins can then be eliminated more easily in the urine.

Carcinogens are toxins that can cause cancer. The way they do this is now fairly well understood. Many carcinogens are known to cause DNA damage. It is now known that this DNA damage occurs in important oncogenes and/or tumor suppressor genes leading to the initial events that cause cancer. Besides damage to DNA, carcinogens can also affect other parts of the cell and alter energy production in a cancer cell.

Common carcinogens include certain industrial and environmental chemicals, asbestos, and ionizing and ultraviolet radiation. Carcinogens also occur naturally in many foods at low levels, but they are more abundant in meats that have been charcoal-broiled or overcooked. Various food additives, such as nitrate preservatives, can be carcinogenic as well. Carcinogens are also known to occur in water, in the air we breathe, and in cigarette smoke.

WHAT ARE THE DETOXIFICATION SYSTEMS THAT PROTECT US AGAINST CARCINOGENS AND TOXIC AGENTS?

There are two major detoxification systems that protect us from carcinogens and toxic chemicals. The first system of detoxification is divided into two major *enzymatic* reactions: Phase I reactions and Phase II reactions.

In Phase I reactions, the molecular structure of the carcinogen is changed by a chemical reaction, which makes the carcinogen less carcinogenic. These reactions (chemical changes) are performed by proteins called *enzymes*. The Phase I system contains many enzymes that perform *oxidations, reductions, hydrolyses,* and *hydroxylations*. These are all terms for the specific type of chemical reaction that takes place. An important Phase I enzyme is called *cytochrome P-450*. This enzyme chemically changes molecules by adding an oxygen atom to them so that they are easily eliminated or made less toxic.

In Phase II reactions, a chemical actually attaches (binds) to the carcinogen in order to help eliminate it from the body. Phase II reactions are called *conjugations*. The primary purpose of this type of detoxification system is to rapidly convert dangerous chemicals to conjugated (bound) forms that are water-soluble and easily excreted from the body. One of the most important Phase II reactions in our body is the conjugation reaction that uses D-glucarate. D-glucarate helps the body remove carcinogens, toxins, and compounds that are no longer needed. D-glucarate is found in fruits and vegetables and is also made in our body from glucose. We will discuss this important process in more detail later.

Phase II detoxifying enzymes include *glutathione S-transferases, glucuronosyl transferases* (UDP-glucuronosyl transferases), and *sulfotransferases*. These enzymes do just what their name implies: they transfer the molecule in their name to the toxic molecule. In other words, they conjugate. This conjugation makes the new compound more water-soluble for easier elimination from the body (see Figure 1). For example, glutathione S-transferases conjugate reactive metabolites of carcinogenic compounds with *glutathione*. Glutathione is a very important compound in our body. It is a small *peptide* that contains three *amino acids*. Amino acids are the building blocks of proteins, and peptides are amino acids chemically linked together to form a larger molecule. Proteins contain many amino acids. UDP-glucuronosyl transferases and sulfotransferases conjugate compounds with glucuronic acid and sulfuric acid, respectively.

The second system of detoxification involves neutralizing (inactivating) *free radicals*, which are potentially toxic compounds that are a by-product of our *respiration* (the use of oxygen to generate energy). Free radicals can be neutralized by enzymatic reactions, by antioxidants produced in our bodies, and by antioxidants found in our food.[8,17] Many phytochemicals, including D-glucarate, also exhibit antioxidant activity in addition to their ability to remove toxins by conjugation.[18] Inadequate levels of these detoxification nutrients can lead to cellular damage and possibly cancer.[17,18] This happens because, instead of being neutralized and eliminated, the toxins are available to damage cellular components.

The liver is the major organ involved in the Phase I and Phase II detoxification of carcinogens, toxins, drugs, and medications, and even compounds made in the body, such as *steroids* and *sterols*. Steroids are hormones that are used to regulate many bodily functions and serve as messengers in our body. Besides the liver, detoxification enzymes are also found in skin tissue, in the respiratory tract, in the digestive tract, and in the urinary tract.

Detoxification by Conjugation
Conjugation with glucuronic acid appears to be the principal conjugation pathway in the tissues of all animal species examined to date.[19] The term given to this specific conjugation reaction with glucuronic acid is *glucuronidation*. Glucuronidation appears to be a very important primary mechanism for detoxifying both compounds produced by the body and environmental compounds. Glucuronidation may also provide detoxification even after Phase I reactions have converted toxic compounds to non-toxic ones. For example, after Phase I enzymatic reactions, carcinogens such as *polycyclic aromatic hydrocarbons*, some *nitrosamines, aromatic amines, heterocyclic amines,* and fungal toxins are eliminated by glucuronidation.[19]

Detoxification by Antioxidants
The human body has several systems for defense against free radicals and other *reactive oxygen species* (another term given to compounds that become toxic after they react in some way with toxic oxygen molecules). The various sys-

Figure 1
Detoxification by Conjugation

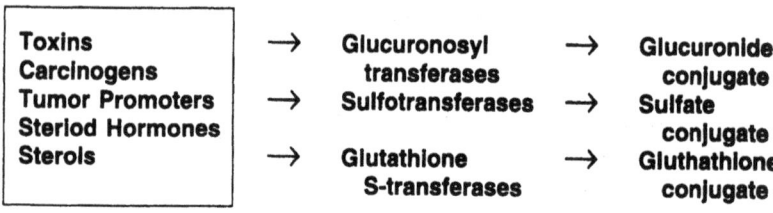

Toxins Carcinogens Tumor Promoters Sterlod Hormones Sterols	$\rightarrow$ $\rightarrow$ $\rightarrow$	Glucuronosyl transferases Sulfotransferases Glutathione S-transferases	$\rightarrow$ $\rightarrow$ $\rightarrow$	Glucuronide conjugate Sulfate conjugate Gluthathione conjugate

tems work together to neutralize different types of free radicals.

One important line of defense is a system of enzymes that include *superoxide dismutase, catalase, glutathione peroxidase, glutathione reductase,* and *thioredoxin reductase.*[8] Superoxide is an oxygen molecule that has become more reactive after the oxygen has oxidized a different substance. The generation of superoxide is a normal physiological process, so we have enzymes that make it non-toxic. The three superoxide dismutases found in the body are enzymes that convert the dangerous superoxide molecule to hydrogen peroxide. Catalase is the enzyme that converts hydrogen peroxide to water and oxygen. Thus, superoxide dismutase and catalase work together to rid the body of the toxic, natural by-products of oxygen metabolism.

Glutathione peroxidases are a family of antioxidant enzymes that contain the micronutrient selenium. These are able to detoxify *hydroperoxides*. Hydroperoxides are similar to hydrogen peroxide except that they are found in *lipids* (cellular membranes). They arise from the reaction of lipids in cell membranes by a process called *lipid peroxidation*. Unsaturated fats are more susceptible to lipid peroxidation compared with saturated fats.

Glutathione reductase and thioredoxin reductase are critical in keeping glutathione and other thiol (sulfur-containing) groups in proteins in a reduced state.[8] The thioredoxin reductase enzyme also contains selenium, and is very important in the synthesis (formation) of DNA. Table 8 gives a summary of some of the antioxidant enzymes.

Table 8
Antioxidant Enzymes

- Superoxide dismutases
- Catalase
- Glutathione peroxidases

- Glutathione reductase
- Thioredoxin reductase

Besides antioxidant enzymes, another line of defense against free radicals are certain chemicals manufactured in the body. These are much smaller than the antioxidant enzymes (which are specialized proteins), but they can help eliminate toxic by-products. Examples of important antioxidants produced in the body that protect us from free radical damage include glutathione, *co-enzyme Q10* (ubiquinol), *lipoic acid*, and *uric acid*.[30]

Vitamins E and C and the carotenoids are good examples of dietary antioxidants that help to protect the human body from free radical damage.[18] Fruits and vegetables provide a valuable source of vitamin C and carotenoids. Since vitamin E is a fat-soluble vitamin, it is abundant in meats, eggs, and butter. Increased levels of dietary antioxidants play a significant role in supporting a person's cellular antioxidant defense system as it works to protect against excessive free radical damage.

However, our body is supposed to maintain a balance between oxidation and reduction. It is important to emphasize that oxidation is a very necessary and important aspect of our life. We all know we breathe oxygen. It is used to generate energy in the cellular organelle called the mitochondria. This is the main energy-producing pathway that drives all the necessary chemical reactions to sustain life. As previously mentioned, the by-products of this process can be damaging to our cells as well. But our bodies have developed elaborate systems, as discussed above, to eliminate the toxic by-products. Antioxidants are thus very important, but there is a growing awareness that the overconsumption of antioxidants may have harmful effects.

GLUCURONIDATION: A MAJOR DETOXIFICATION PATHWAY

Glucuronidation is one of the major detoxification pathways in tissues of all vertebrates. As we said before, glucuronidation is a Phase II reaction in which a highly polar (water-soluble) substance combines with a toxin and carries it out of the body. In this process, carcinogens and tumor promoters bind (conjugate) to the active substance glucuronic acid. Glucuronic acid and carcinogen binding occur primarily in the liver, but can also occur in many other tissues. From the liver, the complex is picked up by bile (which contains waste products) and then carried to the intestines where it is removed in the stool. Alternatively, the complex can pass through the kidneys to be excreted in the urine. Figure 2 shows the detoxification process from glucuronidation. *Glucuronosyl transferase* is the enzyme that performs the conjugation reaction between the carcinogen and glucuronic acid. Table 9 shows some of the carcinogens that are known to be removed from the body by glucuronidation.

Table 9
Carcinogens Known to Be Inactivated by Glucuronidation

- Polycyclic aromatic hydrocarbons
- Various nitrosamines
- Fungal toxins
- Aromatic amines
- Tumor promoters, including steroid hormones
- Heterocyclic amines

Figure 2
Detoxification by Glucuronidation

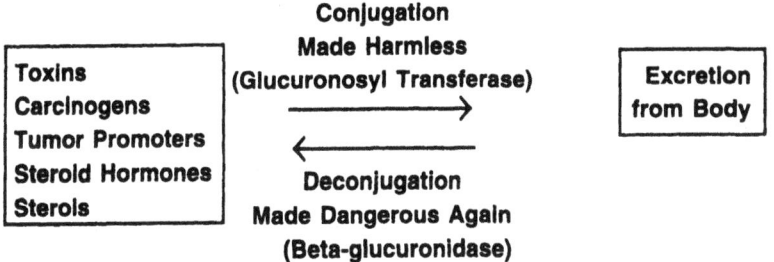

BETA-GLUCURONIDASE: THE BAD ENZYME

An enzyme called beta-glucuronidase reverses glucuronidation. Remember that enzymes are proteins that speed up chemical reactions. Many chemical reactions are reversible, which means the products can change back into the starting material. In this case, beta-glucuronidase reverses the conjugation of compounds that are bound to glucuronic acid, allowing them to go free. Thus, beta-glucuronidase can be considered a "bad enzyme" because it reverses the process that rids the body of carcinogens.

As early as 1957, patients with bladder cancer were identified with elevated beta-glucuronidase activity.[21] Activity of an enzyme is the direct measurement of how fast a reaction is speeded up by the enzyme. Elevated beta-glucuronidase activity suggests that the glucuronidation (detoxification pathway) was reversed in response to bladder cancer, or that the breakdown of conjugates from increased beta-glucuronidase activity stimulated the bladder cancer. Beta-glucuronidase is found in a variety of tissues in the body and promotes the breakdown of glucuronides. This reverses glucuronidation and releases the toxin or carcinogen back into the bloodstream. Some of these reverse-reactions are useful because they "recycle" beneficial compounds, but when carcinogens are recycled into the body, a negative effect from beta-glucuronidase is observed. Elevated beta-glucuronidase levels have been noted following exposure to chemical carcinogens and tobacco smoke in humans. It has also been shown to be elevated in the blood in viral hepatitis, in liver necrosis, and in metastasizing liver cancer.[22] Beta-glucuronidase is elevated in the gastric juices of individuals with gastric cancer.[23] High urinary beta-glucuronidase levels are seen in those with diabetes, bone fractures, and kidney tumors.[24] Tobacco chemicals, carcinogens found in processed foods, certain industrial chemicals, and common and prescribed drugs also increase beta-glucuronidase levels and cause elevated glucuronic acid excretion. Certain food additives found in processed lunchmeat and polycyclic aromatic hydrocarbons in charbroiled meat have also been shown to have this effect.

In a healthy body, detoxification enzymes conjugate (bind) carcinogens to glucuronic acid or sulfuric acid to become a glucuronide or sulfate complex. This makes them water-soluble and easier to eliminate in an inactive form. This is part of the normal detoxification system of the body. In glucuronidation, there is no guarantee that the glucuronic acid conjugated complex will be excreted in the bile. We have already emphasized that if beta-glucuronidase levels are elevated, the carcinogen can be released back into the body. However, in the presence of high levels of D-glucarate, beta-glucuronidase can be inhibited. This process is depicted in Figure 3.

In enzymes, there is a special location called the *active site* where the chemical reaction is speeded up. The compound that is getting chemically altered, or changed, is called the *substrate*. The substrate must bind to this active site in order for the reaction to occur. Number 1 in Figure 3 shows the conjugation of glucuronic acid with an active carcinogen.

Because enzymes have specificity, there is usually only one substrate that gets altered chemically. But sometimes, a different compound, one that is not altered, goes into the active site. When this happens, the substrate cannot react with the enzyme. Number 3 in Figure 3 shows D-glucarate binding to the active site of beta-glucuronidase. This inhibits the reversal of conjugation, and still allows the carcinogen to be excreted from the body. Remember, this happens even in the presence of the "bad enzyme," because the D-glucarate stops deconjugation.

GLUCURONIDATION PROTECTS AGAINST ABNORMAL LEVELS OF STEROID HORMONES

Glucuronidation also rids our bodies of unhealthy levels of hormones such as testosterone, estrogen, and progesterone. Estrogen and progesterone are female hormones produced by the ovaries. They are involved in controlling growth and the events of the menstrual cycle, and in maintaining bone structure. Estrogen in the body occurs in three forms: estrone, estradiol, and estriol. The various forms of estrogen are either conjugated (bound) or free.

Excess levels of the free form of estrogen have been associated with different forms of cancer. The body can remove excess estrogen through glucuronidation. Approximately 90 percent of estrogen is bound with glucuronic acid to form a glucuronide; the rest is bound to a sulfate compound.

Elevated levels of beta-glucuronidase and steroid hormones have also been associated with the incidence of tumor production in the body. It has been shown that as beta-glucuronidase levels rise, estrogen receptors increase in number,[25] and therefore more free estrogen can associate with its receptor. This can cause more breast cell growth and lead to cancer. Men with benign prostate hyperplasia (BPH), which is a condition that results in an enlarged prostate with more cells, also have elevated free estrone and estradiol levels.[26]

IDENTIFYING THE ACTIVE SUBSTANCE IN GLUCURONIDATION

Before the active substance in glucuronidation could be found, researchers had to know more about glucuronic acid. They

Figure 3
D-Glucarate Inhibition of Beta-Glucuronidase
(Enhanced Excretion of Carcinogens and Excess Steroid Hormones)

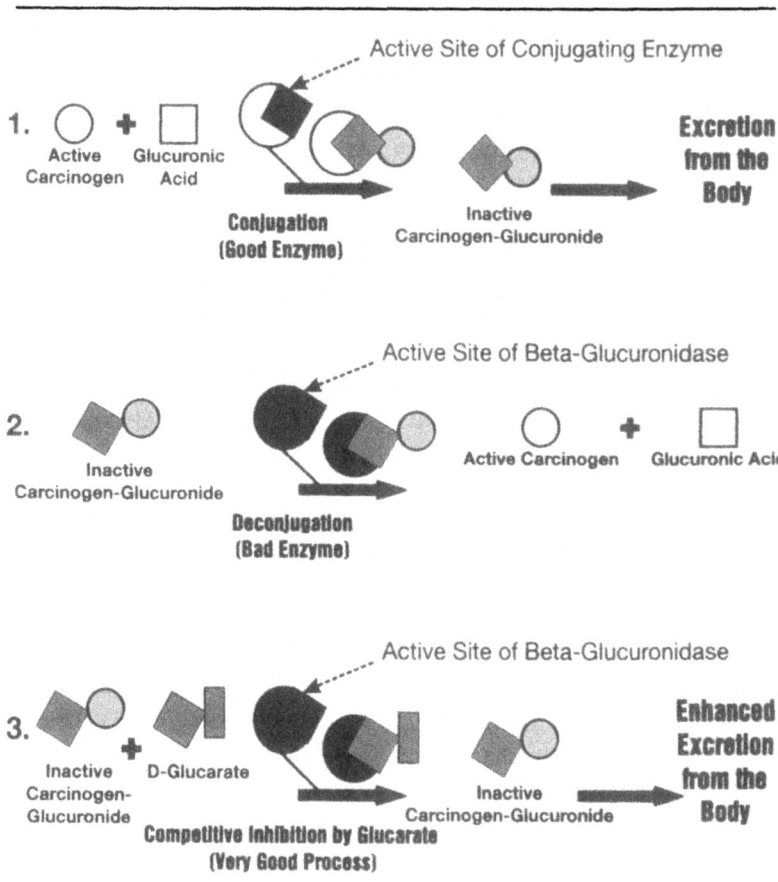

discovered that glucuronic acid can also react to make other related chemical compounds. These other compounds were *D-glucaric acid; D-glucaro-1,4-lactone;* and *D-glucaro-6,3-lactone.*

D-glucaro-1,4-lactone (GL) is very important in glucuronidation. In 1957, GL was recognized as the active substance involved in the inhibition of beta-glucuronidase. This inhibition stops the reversal of glucuronidation (see Figure 3), allowing toxins and carcinogens to be eliminated.

The related compound, D-glucaric acid, is found in foods such as apples, grapefruit, brussels sprouts, and broccoli. It is also found in mung bean seedlings, tomato leaves, and a variety of succulent plants. D-glucurate, as previously discussed, can also be produced in the body from glucuronic acid. D-glucaric acid can be converted to GL in our body.

As D-glucaric acid enters the body, it is absorbed in the gastrointestinal tract and maintained in the bloodstream. It is then transported in the blood to various organs to help in detoxification and is eventually excreted in the bile or the urine.

D-glucaric acid is also elevated after the consumption of caffeine, marijuana, or tobacco[27] which requires increased glucuronidation of chemicals in these substances. The more these substances were consumed, the greater the excretion of D-glucaric acid.

Since GL is the active component in one of our body's most powerful detoxification pathways, it would be extremely therapeutic if it could be administered orally. So, in the 1960s, GL was evaluated using animal experiments. Researchers discovered that it was broken down and excreted quickly from the body when given to the animals orally.

Researchers then began to manufacture analogues (similar chemical compounds) to evaluate their potential use as inhibitors of beta-glucuronidase. The goal of increasing GL levels in the body with an oral supplement was achieved using the compounds calcium D-glucarate and potassium hydrogen D-glucarate. Both were found to be non-toxic.

Since the GL oral supplement was quickly excreted, researchers wanted to find a similar compound that would be retained in the body. Calcium D-glucarate was perfect since it acted as a precursor to GL, and provided the best slow release of this detoxifying agent.

PROTECTIVE CALCIUM D-GLUCARATE

At the University of Texas M. D. Anderson Cancer Center, repeated *in vitro* and animal studies have been performed to demonstrate the effectiveness of calcium D-glucarate.[28] Oral ingestion of calcium D-glucarate has been shown to inhibit beta-glucuronidase. This means the body is better able to get rid of carcinogens and waste products. In one animal study,[29] a single dose of calcium D-glucarate inhibited beta-glucuronidase activity by 57 percent in the blood, 44 percent in the liver, 39 percent in the intestines, and 37 percent in the lungs. In the same study, beta-glucuronidase activity in the microflora was inhibited by 70 percent in the small intestine and by 54 percent in the colon.

Calcium D-glucarate has the greatest potential as a compound against carcinogens for a number of reasons: (1) It is non-toxic when orally administered; (2) it is converted to the active GL form in the body, which inhibits beta-glucuronidase; and (3) it provides for the slow release of GL after ingestion.

In 1994, a study in England demonstrated that calcium D-glucarate did not need to be converted into GL in order to directly inhibit beta-glucuronidase.[30]

A number of dietary supplements look promising in cell culture studies (studies using cells in an incubator), but the human body is not able to absorb the supplements. Calcium

D-glucarate's absorption rates have been studied in rodents with primary mammary cancer,[31] by following its progress through the digestive tract. After the administration of one dose of calcium D-glucarate, the average levels of calcium D-glucarate in the blood of the study animals increased ten times after one hour. After three hours, calcium D-glucarate levels dropped almost 75 percent, and then at fifteen hours, the levels increased beyond the one-hour levels. After twenty-four hours, 38 percent of the calcium D-glucarate was excreted in the urine, while 30 percent remained in the gastrointestinal system. The liver and gastrointestinal tissue had three to four times greater concentration of calcium D-glucarate than in the blood. This demonstrates that orally injested calcium D-glucarate accumulates in these tissues. This suggests that its beneficial effects in our body arise from increased detoxification, since the liver is our primary detoxification organ.

CALCIUM D-GLUCARATE AGAINST CANCER

Calcium D-glucarate appears to inhibit beta-glucuronidase in animals, so that the glucuronidation pathway is not reversed. It also has been shown to have a direct effect on how cells multiply, slowing down the rate that cancer cells grow. In one study, the chemical carcinogen diethylnitrosamine was used to induce liver cancer in rats.[32] Following administration of calcium D-glucarate for five months, liver carcinogenesis was inhibited at the initiation stage. Researchers concluded that calcium D-glucarate had a direct effect on inhibiting carcinogenesis in the liver when the toxic compound diethylnitrosamine was used to induce the cancer.

As previously noted, calcium D-glucarate has been shown

to inhibit cancer during all three stages of the disease: initiation, promotion, and progression. This is one reason calcium D-glucarate is such a good agent for the risk reduction of cancer.

Calcium D-glucarate has also been shown to extend the latency period of carcinogenesis.[33] This is the time prior to the development of the first tumor.

BREAST CANCER

Breast cancer is the second leading cause of cancer death in women. The risk of women developing breast cancer in the United States is 1 in 8. The American Cancer Society has estimated that there will be 180,000 new breast cancer cases in 1999. In addition, approximately 44,000 deaths will occur from this disease. The American Cancer Society predicts that in the United States in 1999 there will be 179,000 new invasive breast cancer cases diagnosed in women and 1,600 among men.[34] Breast cancer risk has also been found to increase with age—more than 77 percent of new cases occur in women over 50. African American women have a greater chance of death from breast cancer (31 per 100,000) than Caucasian women (26 per 100,000).

As we previously discussed, many factors can contribute to breast cancer. Inheritance of oncogenes certainly increases the risk of breast cancer. Environmental factors also play a significant role. These factors include exposure to chemical carcinogens and excess total calorie consumption over a long period of time. Finally, the association between breast cancer and estrogen levels in the blood provides some clues about the increased rates of breast cancer in women as they age. Menopause appears to play some role in breast cancer, which could be related to estrogen or overall hormonal balance. Studies have shown that young women at high risk for breast cancer have an altered estrogen profile compared to control groups.

One study at Creighton University, College of Medicine, looked at thirty young pre-menopausal women at high risk for breast cancer.[35] This study was designed to determine differences in urine steroid levels between healthy women and those considered at high risk for cancer. The control group did not include any first-degree relatives with breast cancer. Both groups were similar in age, height, and weight at first pregnancy. Blood levels of seven hormones were analyzed in both groups. Urine was collected and reacted with beta-glucuronidase to determine the levels of hormones removed by the urine. The only difference found in urinary hormone levels was estrogen: The high-risk group had lower urinary excretion of two forms of estrogen, estrone and estradiol (forms usually found in the body). Both of these hormones are associated with breast cancer. It is possible that these hormones were bound and excreted as a sulfate complex and therefore were not detected in this study as free hormones in the urine. Nonetheless, reduced excretion of these forms of estrogen suggests greater beta-glucuronidase enzyme activity and therefore less glucuronidation. This leads to the theory that breast cancer could be associated with the actual amount of estrogen conjugated and removed from the body through glucuronidation.

A very important step in developing treatments and preventive agents for breast cancer came with the discovery that calcium D-glucarate supplementation increases glucuronidation. This is thought to help reduce excess estrogen levels and carcinogens. Calcium D-glucarate has been shown to inhibit mammary cancer in over twenty animal and *in vitro* studies.

Research studies have shown that calcium D-glucarate inhibits mammary tumor incidence and number.[13,36] In one animal study, supplementation of 2 percent of calcium D-glucarate daily in the diet resulted in a 50 percent inhibition of beta-glucuronidase; blood estradiol levels were reduced 23 percent. Mammary tumor growth during the promotion stage was reduced by 30 percent when calcium D-glucarate was supplemented at 10 percent of the daily diet. There was also a four-fold reduction in the absolute number of tumors in this study.

Calcium D-glucarate has also been shown to be beneficial for mammary cancer when taken in combination with *retinoid*.[31,37] Retinoid is a form of vitamin A that has been successfully tested against cancer in humans and animals. It appears that their combined action somehow works in what we call a *signal transduction pathway*. Signal transduction is a process that cells use to chemically communicate with each other. Sometimes abnormal cellular changes occur in the body that can affect these signals, which may lead to cancer formation. Messages may be sent out to cells that cause them to dedifferentiate and grow out of control. Calcium D-glucarate and retinoid demonstrated a synergistic effect against mammary tumors in animals and human breast adenocarcinoma (cancer) cells tested *in vitro*.[38] Unfortunately, as retinoid dosage levels increase, so does toxicity. Calcium D-glucarate does not pose this problem of toxicity.

In another study from Europe, rats fed calcium D-glucarate and isotretinoin demonstrated an ability to reverse tumor growth. This resulted in a 20 percent decrease in tumor volume.[38] A different study showed a more than 70 percent decrease in mammary tumor development in rats that were given calcium D-glucarate after treatment with carcinogens. Researchers concluded that oral calcium D-glucarate delayed the promotion stage of mammary cancer by lowering estradiol and other precursor steroids.[39]

Calcium D-Glucarate's Effect on Breast Cancer During Different Stages of Carcinogenesis

In 1995, a study was done that looked at calcium D-glucarate's effect on both the initiation and the promotion stages of cancer. The results showed that the replication of breast tumors was reduced by 28 percent during the initiation stage, and reduced by 42 percent during the promotion stage.[33] Inhibition of cancer in the initiation stage is a very important part of calcium D-glucarate's benefit. It lessens the risk that cancer will even start, and therefore makes the promotion and progression stages less likely. Since these are the stages that are more lethal, calcium D-glucarate may be beneficial in reducing overall mortality rates from breast cancer.

Calcium D-Glucarate Reduces Estrogen Receptors

Hormones work as signals in our body. They are the messengers that help regulate our bodily functions. After a hormone is released into the blood and enters into target cells, it binds to its *receptor*, and the chemical signal it carries is given to the cell to which it is bound.

Elevated beta-glucuronidase enzyme activity has been associated with the level of estrogen and progesterone (another hormone) receptors in mammary carcinomas.[28] In a fifteen-week study, mammary cancer in rodents was induced with the carcinogen DMBA. The resulting tumors were allowed to grow to approximately 1 cm in diameter. Calcium D-glucarate supplementation reduced estrogen receptors by 48 percent with a corresponding reduction in tumor growth.[40]

Some studies have suggested that women with fibrocystic disease have a greater risk for breast cancer. Although this risk may include only those who have epithelial hyperplasia (multiple cell reproduction), beta-glucuronidase has been found in cysts. A human study was performed to evaluate beta-glucuronidase levels in breast cyst fluid of patients with fibrocystic breast disease.[41] After the evaluation, participants fell into two groups. Compared to the control group who were outpatients with no history of benign breast disease, one test group contained normal levels of beta-glucuronidase, whereas the other group had three times higher levels than the control. This research study demonstrated that as beta-glucuronidase levels increased, levels of non-conjugated (free) estradiol also increased. More investigation needs to be done to determine if there is any significance direct related to breast cancer, and one such study is now in progress. Calcium D-glucarate is being used in a Phase I trial (first human testing stage) at Memorial Sloan-Kettering Cancer Center with women at high risk for breast cancer. This study is in collaboration with the National Cancer Institute at the National Institutes of Health.[42]

LUNG CANCER

Calcium D-glucarate has been found to be an effective inhibitor of lung cancer in mice induced with the carcinogens benzo(a)pyrene, urethane, and 1-nitropyrene.[13,43] Calcium D-glucarate was also shown to cause a 70 percent decrease in the binding of the carcinogen benzo(a)pyrene to DNA in both the mouse liver and lungs. Benzo(a)pyrene is a potent carcinogen found in cigarette smoke, so these tests suggest that smokers would benefit from calcium D-glucarate supplementation. The researcher Dr. Walaszek and his associates at the AMC Cancer Research Center are presently studying the effect of calcium D-glucarate on various early biomarkers of lung cancer. Similar studies on the effects of calcium D-glucarate on early biomarkers of breast cancer are also under way with special emphasis on high-risk females.

COLON CANCER

Just as breast and lung cancer are very common in the United States, so is colon cancer (colorectal cancer). Approximately 160,000 Americans were diagnosed with colorectal cancer in 1998. Several experimental animal studies have been conducted on the protective effect of calcium D-glucarate against colon cancer induced by various potent carcinogens.[13,44,45] For example, Dwivedi and coworkers used the carcinogen azoxymethane to induce intestinal cancer in rats in a study published in 1989.[46] Calcium D-glucarate supplementation inhibited adenocarcinoma formation when given in the tumor initiation stage and when administered in the promotional stage of cancer. Specifically, their data indicate that calcium D-glucarate significantly inhibited the incidence and size of both intestinal and colon cancers and also reduced the metastatic potential. The controls that used *calcium gluconate* (known to not promote glucuronidation) did not show any inhibitory activity. Furthermore, Yoshimi and coworkers[45] demonstrated that potassium hydrogen D-glucarate was a potent inhibitor of azoxymethane-induced colon cancer in the same rat colon model. Thus, it seems that both calcium D-glucarate and potassium hydrogen D-glucarate have the ability to inhibit the induction of colon cancer in this specific rat model.

In addition, Walaszek and coworkers[14] have reported that calcium D-glucarate and D-glucaro-1,4-lactone (GL) inhibit cell proliferation (growth) induced by carcinogens in the rat colon, rat mammary gland, and mouse skin. Therefore, the inhibition of beta-glucuronidase and inhibition of carcinogen-induced cell proliferation may contribute to the anti-colon cancer effect of D-glucarate.

LIVER AND BLADDER CANCER

Only limited experimental animal data is available on the effects of calcium D-glucarate in liver cancer. In a study using rats treated with diethylnitrosamine and phenobarbital (known carcinogens), calcium D-glucarate was shown to inhibit the induction of pre-neoplastic-altered hepatic foci.[13] Although these altered foci in the liver are not liver cancer, they are recognized as predictive of liver cancer as induced by liver carcinogens. As observed in the breast, lung, and colon, calcium D-glucarate contributes to the detoxification of carcinogens and tumor promoters. And, because the compound has an inhibitory effect on carcinogen-induced cell proliferation in animals, there is a good chance that calcium D-glucarate should be effective against the induction of liver cancer in humans.

As with liver cancer, only limited data can be found on the effect of calcium D-glucarate in bladder cancer. One study, however, on a derivative of D-glucarate, *2,5-di-O-acetyl-D-glucaro-1,4,6,3-dilactone*, showed that it was effective in counteracting bladder cancer that was induced in rats by the carcinogen *2-acetylaminofluorene*.[19] Presently, the mechanism by which this D-glucarate derivative inhibits bladder cancer is unknown. However, investigators agree that a similar

D-GLUCARATE: A NUTRIENT AGAINST CANCER / 37

effect to the calcium D-glucarate inhibition of beta-glucuronidase may be relevant in this study. This suggests that there may be a role for supplemental calcium D-glucarate in reducing the risk reduction of bladder cancer in humans.

SKIN CANCER

Two studies have been reported that looked at the effect of calcium D-glucarate and D-glucaro-1,4-lactone (GL) on skin tumors induced in mice by a polycyclic aromatic hydrocarbon carcinogen and by a phorbol ester tumor promoter. Walaszek[13] reported in the journal *Cancer Letters* that the induction of both papillomas and squamous cell carcinomas in mice were significantly inhibited by calcium D-glucarate supplementation.[14] In another study, Boone and his colleagues[44] reported that both calcium D-glucarate and GL inhibited certain preliminary biomarkers for skin cancer. With the likelihood that one in five Americans will develop some form of skin cancer in their lifetime (approximately one million cases per year), any preventive agent, such as calcium D-glucarate, may be enormously beneficial in reducing the damaging effects of this disease.

PROSTATE CANCER

In preliminary studies, researchers observed that dietary calcium D-glucarate significantly inhibited the growth of rat prostate cancer cells that were transplanted to a host rat that did not already have cancer. In this same animal model, calcium D-glucarate also effectively reduced the levels of a specific tumor marker, suggesting that it has the potential to reduce cancer formation. The inhibition of the growth of the hormone-dependent transplantable rat prostate cancer after the transplant of cancer cells is thought to be from a decrease in steroid synthesis in the these animals. Other studies showed that the growth of human hormone-dependent prostate cancer cells *in vitro* were suppressed by the addition of D-glucaro-1,4-lactone in the culture medium. Although preliminary, these results suggest calcium D-glucarate may be effective against prostate cancer in men. Since approximately 170,000 men will be diagnosed with prostate cancer in the United States in 1999 alone, any possible effective preventive agent, such as calcium D-glucarate, will be extremely important.

SUMMARY OF CALCIUM D-GLUCARATE AND CANCER

The results of various animal studies on calcium D-glucarate's beneficial effects in breast, lung, colon, liver, bladder, and skin cancers suggests that it may also be useful in treatment and for risk reduction of these cancers in humans. Human studies are just now beginning to determine if the results observed in animals are also found in people. Since calcium D-glucarate has no known side effects when injested in moderate doses, its use as a supplement would appear to be ideal for people at risk for cancer.

Table 10 summarizes the protective effect of D-glucarate and derivatives against various cancers in animals and humans.

Table 10
Protective Effect of D-Glucarate and Derivatives Against Various Cancers[47]

• Breast	• Bladder
• Lung	• Skin
• Colon	• Prostate
• Liver	

IS IT SAFE?

It is important to once again state that D-glucaric acid is a natural compound produced in small amounts by mammals and by some plants.[48,49] Calcium D-glucarate and its derivatives have been extensively investigated in long-term animal studies using rats, mice, hamsters, and chickens, with no reported toxic effects at dosages of 0.5 to 10 percent of the diet. A review of all studies to date reveals only beneficial effects.

Furthermore, although only limited human studies have been carried out, no evidence of toxicity has been noted at dosages of 1.5 g per day. As we said before, the National Cancer Institute has initiated a Phase I trial in which calcium D-glucarate is administered to women at high risk for breast cancer.[42] To date, these studies have shown no evidence of toxicity even at the very high dose of 10 grams of calcium D-glucarate per day, and no side effects have been reported.

DIETARY SOURCES OF D-GLUCARATE

The levels of D-glucarate naturally occurring in a variety of fruits and vegetables were determined recently by Walaszek and his associates,[48] who found between 0.1 gram per kilogram and 3.5 grams per kilogram. Table 11 gives a summary of these levels in fruits and vegetables.

HOW MUCH D-GLUCARATE SHOULD BE TAKEN DAILY?

Based on scientific studies performed thus far, you would need to ingest 200 mg to 2,000 mg per day of D-glucaric

Table 11
Amount of D-Glucaric Acid in Various Fruits and Vegetables

Food	Weight in Grams	D-Glucaric Acid Content (g/kg food)	Amount in One Serving (mg)
Apple (whole)	138	2.3	311
Grapefruit (half, pink)	123	3.6	443
Broccoli (raw, chopped, cooked, 1 cup)	156	3.4	530
Alfalfa sprouts (1 cup)	33	3.5	114
Brussel sprouts (cooked, 1 cup)	156	2.7	417
Cherries	145	1.4	207
Apricots (dried halves, 1 cup)	130	1.4	181

acid or its derivatives, in order to obtain the beneficial effects of this compound. (So apparently an apple a day may indeed keep the doctor away!)

Since we do not know for sure how much D-glucarate an individual needs daily to attain maximum protective benefits against various cancers, we can only estimate. Since there is plenty of evidence that an overall reduced calorie diet greatly reduces the risk of developing cancer, it may be important to supplement with calcium D-glucarate, and include a limiting amount of fruit, vegetables, and other food products so that excess calories are not consumed.

WHERE CAN CALCIUM D-GLUCARATE BE PURCHASED?

Besides the natural form of D-glucaric acid found in fruits and vegetables, calcium D-glucarate can be purchased as a dietary supplement in many health food, mass market, and grocery stores throughout the United States. It comes in the form of capsules, tablets, powdered drinks, and health bars. It can also be found in cosmetic products for topical use.

REFERENCES

1. *Diet, nutrition and cancer.* 1982. Washington, D.C.: National Academy of Sciences Press.
2. Slaga, T. J., ed. 1980. *Modifiers of chemical carcinogenesis: An approach to the biochemical mechanism and cancer prevention.* New York: Raven Press.
3. Slaga, T. J. 1980. Food additives and contaminants as modifying factors in cancer induction. In *Nutrition and cancer,* eds. G. R. Newell and N. M. Ellison, 279–90. New York: Raven Press.
4. Doll, R., and R. Peto. 1981. The cause of cancer: Quantitative estimates of available risks of cancer in the United States today. *Journal of the National Cancer Institute* 66:1192–1308.
5. Wynder, E. L., and G. B. Gori. 1977. Contribution of the environment to cancer incidence: An epidemiologic exercise. *Journal of the National Cancer Institute* 58:825–32.
6. International Agency Against Cancer. 1985. *IARC monographs on the evaluation of the carcinogenic risk of chemicals to humans: Tobacco habits other than smoking,* 37. Lyon, France: International Agency Against Cancer.
7. International Agency Against Cancer. 1986. *IARC monographs on the evaluation of the carcinogenic risk of chemicals to humans: Tobacco smoking,* 38. Lyon, France: International Agency Against Cancer.
8. Frei, B., ed. 1994. *National antioxidants in human health and disease.* New York: Academic Press.
9. Steinmetz, K., and J. D. Potter. 1991. A review of vegetables, fruit, and cancer I. *Cancer Causes and Control* 2:325–57.
10. Pryor, W. A. 1992. Antioxidants in the prevention of human atherosclerosis. *Circulation* 85:2337–44.
11. Slaga, T. J., and W. M. Bracken. 1977. The effects of antioxi-

dants on skin tumor initiation and aryl hydrocarbon hydroxylase. *Cancer Research* 37:1631–35.

12. Slaga, T. J. 1995. Inhibition of skin tumor initiation, promotion, and progression by antioxidants and related compounds. *Critical Reviews in Food Science and Nutrition* 5(1& 2): 51–57.

13. Walaszek, Z. 1990. Potential use of D-glucaric acid derivatives in cancer prevention. *Cancer Letters* 54:1–8.

14. Walaszek, Z., et al. 1990. *Procceedings of the American Association for Cancer Research* 31:124.

15. *What you need to know about cancer.* 1988. NIH Publication No. 90-1566.

16. Slaga, T. J., J. DiGiovanni, L. D. Winberg, and I. V. Budunova. 1995. Skin carcinogenesis: characteristics, mechanisms, and prevention. In *Progress in clinical and biological research series—Growth factors and tumor promotion: Implications for risk assessment,* eds. M. McClain, T. J. Slaga, R. LeBoeuf, and H. Pitot, 1–20. New York: Wiley-Liss.

17. Wattenberg, L. W. 1992. Inhibition of carcinogenesis by minor dietary constituents. *Cancer Research* 52:2085–91.

18. Huang, M. T, T. Osawa, C. Ho, and R. T. Rosen, eds. 1994. American Chemical Society Symposium Series 546. *Food phytochemicals for cancer prevention I: fruits and vegetables.* Washington, D.C.: American Chemical Society.

19. Dutton, G. J. 1980. *Glucuronidation of drugs and other compounds.* Boca Raton, Fla.: CRC Press.

20. Ames, B. N., et al. 1993. Oxidants, antioxidants, and the degenerative diseases of aging. *Procceedings of the National Academy of Sciences* 90:7915–22.

21. Boyland, E., et al. 1957. *Enzyme activity relation to cancer.* London: Chester Beatty Research Institute, Royal Cancer Hospital, 578–89.

22. Goldbarg, J. A., et al. 1959. A method for the colorimetric determination of beta-glucuronidase in serum, urine, and tissue assay of enzymatic activity in health and disease. *Gastroenterology* 36:193.

23. Simon, L., and A. Figus. 1972. Diagnostic value of determination of lactate dehydrogenase and beta-glucuronidase activity in gastric juice. *Digest* 7:174.

24. Gonick, H. C., and A. Schapiro. 1967. Urinary enzymes in renal disease. *Clinical Research* 15.

25. Vierbuchen, M., et al. 1985. Die Bedeutung hydrolytischer

enzymaktivitaeten im mammakarzinom. *Verhandlungen Der Deutschen Gesellschaft Fur Pathologie* 69:131.
26. Brochu, M., et al. 1987. Comparative study of plasma steroid and steroid glucuronide levels in normal men and in men with benign prostatic hyperplasia. *Prostate* 11:33–40.
27. Kyle, E., A. Carper, and P. Bowan. 1987. Caffeine consumption and vegetarian diets affect D-glucarate acid excretion in man. *Nutrition Research* 7:461–70.
28. Walaszek, Z., et al. 1990. Antiproliferative effect of dietary glucarate on the Sprague-Dawley rat mammary gland. *Cancer Letters* (Netherlands) 49(1):51–57.
29. Dwivedi, C., et al. 1990. Effect of calcium glucarate on beta-glucuronidase activity and glucarate content of certain vegetables and fruits. *Biochemical Medicine and Metabolic Biology* 43(2):83–92.
30. Curley, R. W. Jr., et al. 1994. Activity of D-glucarate analogues: synergistic antiproliferative effects with retinoid in cultured human mammary tumor cells appear to specifically require the D-glucarate structure. *Life Sciences* (England) 54(18):1299–303.
31. Webb, T., et al. 1994. Pharmacokinetics relevant to the anticarcinogenic and anti-tumor activities of glucarate and the synergistic combination of glucarate/retinoid in the rat. *Biochemical Pharmacology* 347(9):1655–1660.
32. Oredipe, O. A., et al. 1992. Dietary D-glucarate mediated inhibition of initiation of diethylnitrosamine-induced hepatocarcinogenesis. *Toxicity* 74(2/3):209–22.
33. Abou-Issa, H. 1995. Relative efficacy of glucarate on the initiation and promotion phases of rat mammary carcinogenesis. *Anticancer Research* (Greece) 15(3):805.
34. American Cancer Society. 1998. Available from *http://www.cancer.org/ben/info/brstats.ht* (Internet).
35. Fishman, J., et al. 1979. Low urinary estrogen glucuronides in women at risk for familial breast cancer. *Science* 204(4397):1089–91.
36. Abou-Issa, H., et al. 1988. Putative metabolites derived from dietary combinations of calcium glucarate and N-(4-hydroxyphenyl) retinamide act synergically to inhibit the induction of rat mammary tumors by 7,12-dimethylbenzanthracene. *Proceedings of the National Academy of Sciences* 85:4181–4.
37. Webb, T., et al. 1993. Mechanism of growth inhibition of

mammary carcinomas by D-glucarate and the glucaratereti-noid combination. *Anticancer Research* 13:2095–2100.
38. Abou-Issa, H., A. Koolemans-Beynen, T. A. Meredith, et al. 1992. Antitumour synergism between non-toxic dietary combinations of isotretinoin and glucarate. *European Journal of Cancer* 28A(4/5):784–8.
39. Walaszek, Z., M. Hanausek-Walaszek, J. Minton, et al. 1986. Dietary glucarate as anti-promoter of 7,12-dimethylbenz[a]anthracene-induced mammary tumorigenesis. *Carcinogenesis* 7(9):1463–66.
40. Walaszek, Z., E. Flores, and A. K. Adams. 1988. Effect of dietary glucarate on estrogen receptors and growth of 7,12-dimethylbenz(a)anthracene-induced rat mammary carcinomas. *Breast Cancer Research and Treatment* 12:128.
41. Minton, J. P., et al. 1986. Beta-glucuronidaseuronidase levels in patients with fibrocystic breast disease. *Breast Cancer Research and Treatment* 8:217–22.
42. Heerdt, A. S., et al. 1995. Calcium D-glucarate as a chemopreventive agent in breast cancer. *Israel Journal of Medical Sciences* 31:101–5.
43. Walaszek, Z., M. Hanausek-Walaszek, and T. E. Webb. 1986. Dietary glucarate-mediated reduction of sensitivity of murine strains to chemical carcinogenesis. *Cancer Letters* 33:25–32.
44. Boone, C. W., et al. 1992. Screening for chemopreventive (anticarcinogenic) compounds in rodents. *Mutation Research* 267:251–55.
45. Yoshimi, N., et al. n.d. Inhibition of azoxymethane-induced rat colon carcinogenesis by potassium hydrogen D-glucarate. *International Journal of Oncology* In Press
46. Dwivedi, C., et al. 1989. Effects of the experimental chemopreventative agent, glucarate, on intestinal carcinogenesis in rats. *Carcinogenesis* 10:1539–41.
47. Walaszek, Z. 1993. Chemopreventive properties of D-glucaric acid derivatives. *Cancer Bulletin* 45:453–7.
48. Walaszek, Z., et al. 1996. D-glucaric acid content of various fruits and vegetables and cholesterol-lowering effects of dietary D-glucarate in the rat. *Nutrition Research* 16(4):673–81.
49. Marsh, C. A. 1963. Metabolism of D-glucuronolactone in mammalian systems. *Biochemical Journal* 87:82–90.

McDonald, J. S. 1988. Preclinical evaluation of lovastatin. *American Journal Cardiology* 62(15):16J–27J.

Nigro, N. D., et al. 1977. A comparison of the effects of the hypocholesteremic agents cholestryramine and candiciolin on the induction of intestinal tumors in rats by azoxymethane. *Cancer Research* 37:3198–203.

Reddy, B. S., et al. 1974. Fecal bacterial beta-glucuronidase: Control by diet. *Science* 183:416–17.

Sandstad, O. 1993. Urinary D-glucaric acid, a marker substance for microsomal enzyme induction: Methdological aspects, responses to alcohol, and findings in workers exposed to toluene. *Scandinavian Journal of Clinical and Laboratory Investigation* (England). 53(4):327–33.

Slaga, T. J., and J. DiGiovanni. 1984. Inhibition of chemical carcinogenesis. In *Chemical Carcinogens*, ed. C. E. Searle, vol. 2, 1279–1321. American Chemical Society Monograph, no. 182. Washington, D.C.: American Chemical Society.

Steele, V. F., et al. 1990. Inhibition of transformation in cultured rat tracheal epithelial cells by potential chemopreventive agents. *Cancer Research* 50:2068–74.

Walaszek, Z., et al. 1986. Inhibition of N-methyl-N-nitrosourea-induced mammary turmorigenesis in the rat by a beta-glucuronidase inhibitor. *IRCS Medical Science* 14:677–8.

Walaszek, Z., et al. 1989. Reducton in vivo of the inappropriate levels of endogenous and environmentally-derived compounds by sustained-release inhibitors of beta-glucuronidase. United States Patent #4,845,123.

Walaszek, Z., et al. 1991. Hypocholesterolemic and antiproliferative effects of glucarate. *FASEB Journal* 5:A930.

Walaszek, Z., et al. 1997. D-glucaric acid as a prospective tumor marker. In *Methods in molecular medicine, vol. XX: Tumor marker protocols,* ed. M. Hanausek and Z. Walaszek. Totowa, N.J.: Humana Press Inc.

Walaszek, Z., et al. 1997. Metabolism, uptake, and excretion of a D-glucaric acid salt and its potential use in cancer prevention. *Cancer Detection and Prevention* 21(2):178–90.

Walaszek, Z., M. Hanausek-Walaszek, and T. E. Webb. 1984. Inhibition of 7, 12-dimethylbenzanthracene-induced rat mammary tumorigenesis by 2, 5-di-O-acetyl-D-glucaro-1, 4:6, 3-dilactone, an in vivo beta-glucuronidase inhibitor. *Carcinogenesis* 5(6):767–72.

Walaszek, Z., M. Hanausek-Walaszek, and T. E. Webb. 1988. Repression by sustained-release beta-glucuronidase inhibitors of chemical carcinogen-mediated induction of a marker oncofetal protein in rodents. *Journal of Toxicology and Environmental Health* 23:15–27.

Wattenberg, L., M. Lipkin, C. W. Boone, and G. J. Kelloff, eds. 1992. *Cancer prevention.* Boca Raton, Fla.: CRC Press.

Wilking, N., E. Isadsson, and E. von Schoultz. 1997. Tamoxifen and secondary tumors: An update. *Drug Safety* 16(2):104–17.

Lightning Source UK Ltd.
Milton Keynes UK
UKHW021018130222
398598UK00005B/150

9 780879 839529